Workout Plan

20 Things You Should Be Doing Before and After Every Workout to Achieve Maximum Results

I0417042

Dean Lacy ©2015

About the Author

Dean Lacy has predominantly been working as a personal trainer for the past twenty years and has worked with a variety of personal clients in the health and leisure industry, in fitness gyms and has worked closely with boxing and martial arts clubs. Dean is obsessed with living a long and healthy life.

Dean recently joined the Health Refinement team dedicated to the world of health. Health Refinement are helping to improve people's knowledge of nutrition, fitness, lifestyle and supplements by supplying you with the latest health news, articles, blogs, videos and books. Refining people's minds and bodies to achieve maximisation of health and fitness.

www.healthrefinement.com

Contents

Important Legal Disclaimer:

The information in this book reflects the author's opinions. The author has made every effort to supply accurate information in the creation of this book. The author offers no warranty and accepts no responsibility for any injury or damage of any kind that may be incurred by the reader as a result of actions arising from the use of content in this book. You should consult your medical professional prior to undertaking any exercise regimes and any information from this book should be used under the guidance of said professional. The reader assumes all responsibility for the use of the information provided in this text.

Introduction

There are many different reasons why people might choose to start a good workout routine. Some people love the way that it makes them feel and look and so they will make it a priority to get to the gym as much as possible. Others know that it is good for their health so they will go in order to prevent or treat a disease that they have. Still others will be more interested in losing weight because they do not like the way that they look or feel at their current weight. No matter the reason that you decide to go hit the gym and get in a good workout, it is important that you do the right things before and after to ensure that you are getting the very best workout and not ruining all of the effort that you put into it.

Often you will go to the gym and work out hard just to find that you are not seeing any of the results that you want. You might not be losing the weight that you want, able to work out hard enough, or getting more injuries than you imagined. This can often be because the routine that you have both before and after hitting the gym is going to influence the way and how hard you are able to work out.

Chapter 1 is going to spend some time exploring some of the things that you can do in order to get prepared to go to the gym. It is not always as easy as just putting on the clothes and shoes and then just showing up at the gym, although this is certainly a part of the process. You also need to make sure that you are getting enough hydration, eating the right foods, finding motivation, and stretching beforehand to. These are just a few of the tips that you will find in the first chapter that will help to prepare and motivate you to reach the success that you want before you even get to the gym. They will also help you to get in an amazing work out while you are there.

Chapter 2 skips ahead to when you are done at the gym. While you have already done a lot of work in order to get your body is amazing shape while you were at the gym and you followed the steps that were offered in the first chapter, there is still plenty that you will be able to do once the work out is done. Your body is going to need some help with getting through the recovery process. This process is important because it allows the muscles to heal and feel so much better so you can keep up with the work out. You will learn such great tips as taking some rest, doing light movements to get circulation going, staying hydrated, and even getting a nice relaxing massage after a workout just to name a few. If you go through these steps correctly, you will be amazed at how quickly your muscles can relax and recover without having to take medication or do other things that are not natural in order to keep up with the routine.

Doing the right things before and after your work out are essential to making sure that you get in the best work out that you can and that all of the hard work you put in does not go to waste. Check out the great tips that are offered in this guidebook and get in the best shape of your life in no time!

Chapter 1: Things to Do Before the Workout

Getting a good workout in is critical for so many aspects of your health. It can help you to lose weight, feel better, lose inches around your waist, and there are many health conditions that can be prevented or even reversed when you are able to get in a good workout on a regular basis. But if you are doing things in the wrong way, such as not providing your body with enough nutrition before the workout, you could be working extra hard without seeing any of the benefits. This chapter is going to spend some time on the most important things you should do before hitting the gym to ensure that you are getting the very best out of your workout routine.

Eat Right

The first thing that you will need to do before you go out and hit the gym is make sure that you are eating right. This should be something that you are doing all of the time because your body needs a lot of healthy foods in order to keep going and running at its very best. But about an hour before you go to the gym you should be really watching the foods that you are taking into your body. This is a critical time because the food you eat during this time is going to give you the energy that is needed in order to keep going during the workout.

There is a big debate trying to determine if it is a good idea to eat before a workout or if you should avoid eating until you are done. While the amount that you should consume before you go and workout is going to pretty much depend on the amount that your body needs, it is important that you get enough sustenance before the workout so that you have energy and are not hungry.

It is important that you do not go to a workout with an empty stomach. This might seem like a good idea before you start, but it is going to make it so that you do not have the energy that you need for a good workout and in some cases you may feel like you are sick. A good thing to do is make sure that you eat a small meal or snack about an hour before you decide to workout. Pick a meal or a snack that is high in protein and carbs so that you can have enough energy to keep going. Some good idea for this would include bananas and peanut butter, toast and peanut butter, and Greek yogurt.

Hydration

Hydration is an important part of your workout whether you are thinking before, during, or after the workout. Water is important to getting your body hydrated and ready for the intense workout that you are about to go through. Most people will wait until they are starting to get thirsty during the workout in order to replenish their supply, but it is better for the body if you are able to start hydrating before the workout even begins. This allows the body to have the water that it needs to be intense and can prevent you from getting overheated or dehydrated if you are not able to replenish the water quickly enough.

For the most part, a glass of water before the workout is going to be enough to get the workout going, but if you feel like you need more that is fine. You want to be on the line of being well-hydrated without taking in too much and feeling bloated or too full to do the workout. But if you are doing a really intense workout you might want to consider drinking a couple of glasses to get started and then replenishing as you need.

Most people will feel like they cannot get enough water into their diet because it is too bland and tasteless. It is possible to find waters that have a little bit of flavor or to make infused waters that have the taste and nutrients of fruit in them. These can count as your pre-workout drinks as long as you make sure that the variety you choose does not have a ton of sugar. This sugar is not going to help you to get hydrated like you need before the workout. You should also make sure to avoid the energy drinks on the market. These might be able to provide you with the electrolytes that you need for the workout, but they come with a lot of other things that can harm your body.

Getting Dressed

This might sound like a silly thing to put on the list, but it is actually very important that you get up and get dressed as well as you get dressed in the right clothes that are going to help your workout rather than making it very inefficient. To start with, once you get dressed in your gym clothes, it is much harder to convince yourself that it is not a good idea to go to the gym. This can sometimes be all of the motivation that you need in order to get off that couch and then get to the gym like you should.

It is also important that you take the time to find the right kinds of workout clothes that will help you to get the most out of the exercise. Before you go out the door to the gym, you should make sure that the gear you are wearing is comfortable as well as good for the needs of your family. For starters, pick out shorts and shirts that are breathable. For women, the tanks and the sports bras that you are wearing should give you enough support for the activity at hand; if you are running around and jumping a lot you do not want to be wearing a bra that is not able to help out with that. Also, material that is stretchy is great because it allows you to have a lot of movement when you work out. This is a good thing because it will let you extend and push the muscles as much as you need during the exercise without harming the fabric or making it difficult to move around like you need.

Another option that you need to watch out for are shirts that are moisture wicking. Some options, such as cotton, are going to trap in the sweat which will make it very difficult to cool down like you need to during the workout. But the shirts with moisture wicking will be able to help you cool down as you are going through the whole exercise. There are several brands that offer shirts that would fit this category and you will be able to get them for a pretty reasonable price.

Outside of having the right kinds of comfort in the clothes you pick out for the gym, you also want to pick out an outfit that is going to be able to help you with preventing injuries from working out for the long term. For example, the shoes you pick out are very important. If they do not have the right kind of support that you are looking for, you might find that your knees and heels are more likely to sustain an injury. When you are really interested in getting some good workouts in, you should invest in a good pair of shoes. These will provide you with the support and help that you need in order to get a good workout without the worries of injuries.

While you do not have to pick out special workout clothes and you do not have to spend a lot on the attire that you are wearing, it is still important to pick out the clothes that you want to wear with some care. You can pick out some of the clothes that you already have, but make sure that they are comfortable, that you will be able to move around freely in them, and that they are going to allow you to not get an injury in the process.

Stretch Out

Before any type of workout, whether you are doing weights, making it a really intense cardio day, or you are taking it easy, you should make sure that you are getting some good stretches into the routine. Most people will find that it is easier to skip this phase because they are so excited to just get into the workout and see the results. But there are so many injuries that can happen if you do not make sure that the muscles are warmed up and nice and loose before getting into the main workout. You are still able to get in some good calorie burn during the warm up, plus you will find that it is much easier to do the moves and burn more calories during the main workout if you take some time to do good stretches before hitting the gym.

There are a lot of benefits that you will be able to get when you decide to implement a good workout routine. First off, you will find that a good stretch before working out is able to relax the muscles, making it easier to move around compared to if you didn't stretch and the muscles were tight. In addition, you will find that a good stretch will decrease the chance you have of getting an injury such as tearing, or pulling a muscle. Most of the time people will get an injury when they are working out because they did not take just five minutes or so in order to warm up those joints and muscles and get them ready for the workout.

There are many different exercises that you can do in order to stretch out the body. Some of the most common because they open you up to being prepared for a lot of different exercises includes torso twists, hip openers, ankle rolls, and quad stretches. Depending on the type of exercises you plan to be doing for the workout, you might want to spend some time concentrating on some of the other parts of the body. Some other options might be the shoulder, side, and back stretches because they can help with preventing injuries as well. Make sure that during the stretching you do not push too hard. You want to just warm up the muscles and the joints in order to get ready for a good workout rather than making it so that you work out too much and causing more injuries.

Get Your Head Ready

Half of the work that you will be doing for all of this is getting your head into it. If you can be in the right frame of mind before showing up to the gym, you will find that it is much easier to get up and do the good workout that you would really love. On the other hand, if you do not feel the motivation or the want to go to the gym, you might find that you will not even make it to the gym. Even if you do make it to the gym, the workout that you do is not going to be that great, you are not going to be burning the energy or calories that you would like, and you might cut out of the gym early because you just do not want to put in the work. If you want to get the best workout that you can, it is important that you make sure your mind is in the right frame.

While taking the time to stretch and being physically ready for the workout is important, you need to make sure that you are mentally prepared for the workout before you go to the gym. You will need to find some good ways in order to achieve the motivation and get the inspiration that you need before you go to the gym.

One thing that you can do is find a song or two that is able to pump you up and get you ready for the workout that is coming. You should look through the playlist that you have or online to find just the right song. You can then play this song and let it get you all pumped up before you go to the gym. When you have the right motivation to get started, you are more likely to work out harder and get the better results.

Review the Workout

There are many different workouts that you can choose to do in order to get the right look that you are going for. Whether you are using an app or you are just making it up as you go for what you like to do or even choosing to do a group of workout videos that tell you what to do, it is important that you understand what is expected from you each time that you go and hit the gym. You should know what you should do in terms of the sets, reps, weights, how long you will wait between each one, how long you will interval train, which machines you would like to do and so much more. Know everything that you plan to do on the workout.

This is going to help you in many different ways. First, it can help you to have the motivation to get to the gym. You know ahead of time what you should be doing so you can use this to kind of guilt trip yourself into getting in a good amount of work at the gym. It can also help you because you are going to be able to prepare better mentally when you know ahead of time what to do. You can prep yourself on the ride over to the gym in order to get there and be ready. In addition, when you know what you will be doing on your work out, it will save a lot of time. You will not have to look up and down at the itinerary to figure out what you will be doing because it is already in your head. This could save you a lot of time at the gym and ensures that you are ready to go.

Make a Playlist

Many people will choose to make a good playlist before they go to the gym. They will put on some of their favorite songs to listen to on the go and this can help them get one of the best workouts that they can ever have. There are a lot of benefits that you will be able to get out of making a playlist. Some of these benefits include:

- Pumping you up—when you hear some of your favorite songs while working out, you are more likely to be able to pump yourself up ahead of time. You can turn on the playlist while you are getting dressed and then keep it going all throughout the warm up, the work out, and even the cool down. The constant stream of upbeat music, or whatever is your favorite, can sometimes keep you going better than anything else.

- Keeping you focused—putting the headphones in and listening to some music can make it easier to stay focused the way that you need in order to get the workout done. Sometimes, it is easy to get distracted at the gym. You might run into an old friend or someone else who wants to talk for a bit and then you will slow down or stop the workout completely. You could find something interesting on the TV and then you will not notice that the workout is slowing down. You would be amazed at how many things are able to take your focus and make it difficult to get the good workout that you are looking for. When you listen to music, others will leave you alone and you will find that the workout is much more intense than you could imagine.

- Make time faster—when you have something to concentrate on other than the workout, you are much more likely to keep the focus and attention on that one thing. This is a great way to keep up the work. When you are concentrating on the hard work that you are doing, it is going to feel so much more intense than it really is. When you are focusing on the music instead, you might not notice how hard the workout is and you might go harder than you did in the past.

- Makes the workout fun—who doesn't like to spend time listening to music while they are working out. It can be a lot of fun to listen to your tunes and maybe dance along with them a little bit, which can be a good workout on its own as well. Pick out some of the songs that you like to listen to and it is amazing how much more you are able to get done while also having some fun in the process.

While listening to music is often the best option for you to do in order to get pumped up and get in a good workout, you can also make other choices when it comes to things that you can listen to. Some people like to get books on tape to listen to while they go. This can be a nice alternative because it allows you to still listen and focus on something other than the workout so you can go hard without hardly noticing it.

When you are picking out the music that you want to listen to, you should pick based on your own needs. Most people will pick something that is upbeat and fun so that they are able to keep pace with it and keep going for the workout. But if there is a type of music that you like to listen to better, that is fine. Just pick out a playlist that will last for your whole workout and which is going to keep you motivated and going for the whole time.

Try a Foam Roller

Yes, this one might sound like it is a little bit strange, but it can really help to get you ready before going into an intense work out so it is worth your time to try out. Think about this for a second. Some of your favorite athletes will have some deep tissue specialists come and do some work on them ahead of a practice or the big game. Have you ever wondered why this might be? This is because the treatments that are provided by these specialists are able to break up the knots that are in tissue, increase mobility, and improve the quality of the muscles. This makes it easier for the athlete to get up and get things done when it is the right time.

Of course, you probably do not have a professional who is on call and ready to help you out at any time that you want. But this does not mean that you will not be able to get some of the great effects that you are looking for with a different method.

Take out an old foam roller that you have lying around the house and just use it for about ten minutes; this is all that you will need before you start to see some of the great benefits that you are looking for. Sit down on the floor and make sure that your legs are laying so that they are straight out. Place this foam roller underneath the calf of one leg. Use a medium pressure in order to guide it over the body so that it is able to go over the calf muscle about 8 times. When that is done you can switch it to the other calf and complete the same steps. Keep doing this all up the body and if you run into a spot that is extra tight, make sure to spend a few extra minutes on this. Soon you will notice that all of the tension in your body is gone and you are more ready than ever to get going on your new workout.

One thing to keep in mind when using this method is that you must be careful about where you are using it. It is never a good idea to use it in some sensitive places such as your lower back or on the joints that are on the back of your knees. While you might think that these are good places to put the pressure, you will actually end up causing more harm than good when you begin to do this and you could cause an injury in the process.

Find a Friend

Working out on your own can sometimes be really boring. Going to the gym and just staring at a wall or listening to your music on your own will soon catch up to you, especially if you are a naturally social person. This is when having a friend available can make all of the difference. They will be able to meet you at the gym, keep you motivated, keep you on task, and can even make it more likely that you will show up to the gym.

One of the best ways that you can get going at the gym is to have a friend who is available to help you out. Here are some of the benefits that you will get when you find a workout buddy or a friend who is willing to help you out:

1. More workouts—when you have someone who is by your side and doing the work with you, you are much more likely to do it as well. Often it is easy to convince yourself to skip out on the gym because it is just not that important and no one is going to notice when you are on your own. But if you have someone at the gym who is waiting for you, you might feel a little bit bad if you abandon them in order to just sit on the couch and watch your favorite show again. When you have someone to motivate you, it is much more likely that you will get to the gym and that you will get a good workout in more often.

2. Motivation—you and your workout partner will be able to keep each other motivated. Everyone has those hard days where they just do not want to do the work. But when you have someone else there who is going to be your cheerleader and who makes sure that you are working out to your very best, it is much easier to get to the goals that you have set.

3. Harder workouts—it can become almost like a competition when you are doing a workout with another person. You will be looking to see how well you are doing with another person beside you, but when you are on your own, you might not care and you may have a few times when you just sit back and not work out as hard as you should. You and the other person will be able to push each other and you may find that you are doing a better workout than you were ever able to do all alone.

4. More fun—it is always more fun to do things when you have someone else there to talk to, laugh with, and to get the work done. When you are on your own, it can sometimes be difficult to get the work done because you are just bored or because you feel like it does not matter anyway. But when you have someone else who is there by your side and willing to help out, you would be amazed at how great the workout can be.

As you can see, there are many benefits that you will be able to get if you can just find someone who is willing to work out with you. The two of you will be able to work together in order to get the results that you are looking for and you will love the new friendship bond and time together that you are both getting.

Set Goals

You should always have some kind of goals in place so that you are able to know when you are getting something accomplished or not. If you just go to the gym each day without any idea of what you are doing or if you are actually doing something. When you have a goal in place, you can tell if you are heading in the right direction or if you need to work harder in order to get it all accomplished. Make sure that the goals you are going for are realistic and that you will actually be able to accomplish them with a little hard work.

Setting goals for your workouts is not something that has to be all that difficult. If you just think about the things that you want to accomplish for the workout it can be easy. You might be going to the gym in order to lose weight, to improve your overall health, to get fit, or just to be healthier. No matter what the reason might be, you will want to make sure that you are keeping track of the progress you are making. Of course, you should pick a long term goal that you want to go with and then split it up into smaller goals that are more manageable over time. The smaller goals will help you to see that you are getting somewhere with the work you are doing, but they are easier to do than just working toward the bigger goal.

As you can see, there are a lot of things that you should make sure to do before you decide to go to the gym. While you might have missed out on some of these things in the past before going to the gym, you will find that your motivation and your work out are going to be so much better when you begin to employ some of these tricks. Take a look through them in order to learn more and get ready to be in the best shape of your life.

Chapter 2: Things to Do After a Workout

Now that you have gotten yourself motivated to go to the gym and spent all of that time getting in the best workout that you can at the gym, it is time to make sure that you do the right things after the workout. If you just go home at the end of the work out without the proper routine, you could end up hurting your body, causing yourself some injury, and ruin all of the work that you put in. This chapter is going to spend some time looking at the best things that you can do after a workout to ensure that you are on the right track to the most success and to looking your very best.

For the most part, these things are important because they aid you in getting the right recovery that your body needs. If you just go home and sit on the couch when you are done, your body has not gotten the right cool down or nutrients that it needs in order to feel its very best. Plus you will find that if you do not do the proper recovery process, you might eat too much or not eat the foods that you need in order to keep the weight off and make the work out do what you need. Here are some of the ways that you will be able to recover after a work out to get the best out of the work out and everything you have done so far.

Drink Plenty of Fluids

Of course, you should have been doing this through the whole process as well as before you started the work out or got to the gym, you still need to take some time to refill on the fluids before you take a break from the workout. You will find that after a tough workout, you have lost a lot of the fluid that was in your body. While you should be trying to replace some of it while you are working out so that you do not become dehydrated or light headed, you will also need to take in some after the workout in order to help out with the recovery. Even if you did a good job with getting a lot of water during the workout, you will find that your body is still working hard and the heart is pumping fast so you will still be burning some calories.

Water is important because it is able to support all of the nutrient transfer and metabolic function in the body and if you get the amount of water that is needed after a workout, you will be able to improve the way that the body is able to function. If you are an athlete or you are doing a really intense workout, you will find that the replacement of fluids is going to be the even more critical for you because of all the sweat you will be going through. Make sure that you are able to replace the fluid that is lost from the workout.

A good way to make sure that you are getting enough fluid after a workout is to weigh yourself. Get on the scale ahead of the workout so that you can determine how much you weigh beforehand. Then you can go through and do the workout that you want. Once you are done, you can weigh yourself again. If you weigh less at the end of the workout than you did at the beginning, you should make sure to replace that much weight loss with the water. This weight loss is going to be because of the sweat you went through and would not be because of the calories burned until later on. Drink at least this much water to be replenished and you will be amazed at how much faster you will be able to recover after the workout.

Eat Good Foods

After a hard workout, you will need to make sure to give the body the nutrients it needs in order to refuel and recover the way that you want. After getting in that hard work, your muscles and other body parts would have gone through a lot of the nutrients that you may have taken in earlier in the day. But even after the work out, your muscles and bones are going to be working hard in order to recover and they will need the right nutrients in order to get through this recovery process. This means that if you want the body to recover the way that they should, you will need to take in the right kinds of nutrients after the workout is done. This does not mean that you should leave the gym and go have a big milkshake or a bunch of donuts, but rather that you should take the time to eat healthy and wholesome foods that will give you a lot of healthy nutrients for the best results.

The more exercise that you do, the more important it is that you get the nutrients into your body as soon as possible. This can be the most important if you are working on endurance exercises each day or you are working on getting more muscle into the body. Of course, you can still work on it when you do cardio, but it is most important with the harder intensity exercises. It is ideal if you are able to eat the food within an hour after the workout. Include some foods that contain complex carbs as well as protein.

If you are stuck on ideas of what you should eat after a workout, take a look at this list to help you pick a good snack for your needs:

- Protein shake—a shake is a good way to get in the nutrients that your body needs to be healthy. You should make it with some hemp seeds, almond milk, a little bit of healthy and safe protein powder, and a little bit of banana. This will get you some of the carbs as well as the protein that your body needs after the workout.

- Salad with chickpeas

- Vegetables with some tofu—the tofu will give you the protein that your body needs while the vegetables will be great for the other nutrients that your body needs to be in its best form.

- Quinoa with black berries and pecans

- 2 slices multi grain or whole grain bread with some peanut butter

- Burrito with some brown rice, salsa, and guacamole

These are some great options that will give you the protein, complex carbs, and other nutrients that your body needs in order to get through the recovery process in the most efficient method possible.

Do a Few Stretches

Stretching is not only important before you get started on a workout, it is also important when you are all done with the work out, especially if it is really intense. You will find that after the work out, your muscles are sore and tired from all of the hard work you put them in. If you just go home after doing all of this, the muscles will not have time to cool down and get back to normal. They might tighten up and cause some pain and more likelihood of injury than if you just spent a little bit on stretching. You do not have to spend a ton of time on the stretching part, but just a few minutes will give the muscles a chance to cool down and get ready for the recovery stage.

You can use a lot of the same stretches that you did before the work out, just make sure that you are safe and doing them correctly. The point here is to not push your muscles here too hard; you have already pushed them pretty hard in the warm up and the actual work out so that part is done. The point is that you are working on cooling down the muscles, keeping them from getting tight, and making sure that they have a little rest before stopping in order to prevent injuries. Just a few simple stretches in the area that you did the exercises for the best results.

Get Your Rest

There is nothing that is better for some tired muscles than giving them some rest. It is not a good idea to spend too much time at the gym because you could end up overdoing it on the work out and causing some injury to the muscle group or other parts of your body. It is best for you to just spend about an hour or so at the gym and if you plan to go back the next day, you should make sure that you are working out other parts of the body instead of just causing wear and tear on the same muscle. You need to make sure that you are resting the muscle group that you just did so that it can go through the right recovery process.

While that is important, you do need to make sure that you are also resting the whole body, whether this means taking some time off from the gym to recover or making sure that you are getting enough rest for your body each night. Both are just as important as the other and if you are skipping out on one or the other, you will find that you are not getting the recovery that you need.

Time is the best thing that you can do in order to recover or heal when you are going through an intense work out. Your muscles are not always going to be able to keep up with the things that you are throwing at it and if you do not get some rest, you may find that the body is not able to work as well as before or that you are getting harmed and injured more often. Your body does have a great talent of being able to take care and heal itself, but you have to give it the time to do this. When you rest and wait for a bit after going through a really hard work out, you will find that the natural pace of recovery and repair in the body is going to be much more efficient than anything else that you are able to do on your own. While there are some other things that you can do in order to promote the recovery process in the body, often doing nothing and just giving the body some time will be the best and easiest thing that you can do.

In addition, any time that you get sick or an injury, you will need to take some extra time to heal and get better. While this can be difficult to give up the gym time, especially if you have a hard time with staying motivated or if you are really close to reaching your goals, you will need to do this. If you go back to the gym and your intense workouts before your body is ready, you will find that your body is more likely to go through another injury or to worsen the one that you already have. Just give your body the rest and relaxation that it needs and you will be amazed at how much better you are able to perform later on.

Try Out Active Recovery

If you are taking a day off from the work outs that you have been doing, you might want to practice doing some active recovery. This is a good way to keep the body moving a little bit without going too intense. You will still be able to get moving without working out too intensely and harming the muscles during their recovery time. Some people believe that doing some easy and gentle movements will be able to promote circulation. When you have good circulation to the muscles and other parts of the body, you will be able to promote nutrients getting to the muscles while also removing any waste that is produced when you do the workouts. If you are able to do these gentle movements on your off days, it may be able to help you to refuel and repair the body more effectively than just sitting there all day long after a workout.

When you are doing this, you need to make sure to take it slow. You are not really doing a full workout and most likely will not even get the heart to beat that fast. You are simply working to move the muscles a bit to keep circulation going and the muscles ready to recover. This is going to be more like a stretching period than a full workout and could be as simple as getting up and walking around the block a few times or doing some simple stretches that just move the blood and nutrients around a bit.

Massage

Most people will love the sound of this one. Who wouldn't love to have an excuse to get out and have someone give them a nice relaxing massage, especially when they are done with an intense workout that has left them worn and tired? Massage is important because it not only feels good, it can help you to relax and improves the circulation that you will need to get to the muscles after they get tense and tired. Let's look at all of these benefits together.

- Feels good—when something feels good, you will be able to relax a bit more. This can help you to get the rest that your body needs after you go through the work out and the muscles are more likely to recover.

- Relaxed—you will find that after the work out, you will be a bit tense and maybe even a bit jittery. This is because the adrenaline and the blood pumping is going to keep you awake and ready to go through anything. When you have a massage after the work out, you can get the muscles to relax a bit and not be so tense. You will also be able to get the rest of your body to calm down and just get some of the rest that you need.

- Nutrients to the muscles—your muscles need to have the time to relax and get the nutrients that it needs in order to recover. If the circulation of the blood is not able to get into the muscles, there is no way that you will be able to get in the nutrients that it needs. You can make sure to relax a bit and get those nutrients into the muscles where they belong.

If you are able to find someone to do the massage, you will most likely be able to get the most relaxation out of the process. You will not have to do the work or worry about it and you can just concentrate on getting the relaxation that you need after the work out. You can find a loved one or go to a professional in order to get it done. On the other hand, if you do not have someone on hand who is able to help you get the massage that your body needs, you can still do some self-massage techniques such as using the foam roller that was mentioned in the beginning chapter of this book.

Try Hot and Cold Therapy

A great way for you to get what your body needs in order to stay healthy, strong, and ready for the next work out, is to help your muscles recover using hot and cold therapy.

There are a lot of athletes and others who work out really intensely who swear that a good ice bath is able to help you to recover after a workout. This, they say, not only helps recovery, but it will help with preventing injuries in the muscles and joints as well as reducing the amount of soreness felt in the muscles.

Of course, this is a rather extreme approach and not something I would encourage without professional medical guidance.

This is when you could use another therapy known as contrast therapy; this is a therapy that will have you using alternating cold and hot temperatures. You could try hot and cold showers/baths but using compresses is a safe and handy alternative. Ice and heat packs are an easy way of creating a similar result and these packs can be kept at home or carried out in your bag/car.

The theory behind this is that continually dilating and constricting the blood vessels will remove and flush out any of the waste products that might be lingering in the tissues. If this waste material is not removed, it can continue to build up in the muscles, preventing the nutrients from getting in, and causing some damage and potential injury during recovery. In addition, there has been some research done that shows that when using the contrast therapy, you might be able to reduce DOMS or delayed onset muscle soreness.

Sleep

With all of the hard work that you have been putting in to getting healthy and making sure that you are getting the best work out at the gym that you possibly can, it is important that you are also getting the amount of sleep that your body needs. Many people will work out hard and then stay up late to get things done and then be up early the next day for work or for school. While this might be the way that a lot of people live their lives because they are so busy, it is not a good way to go through the recovery that your muscles and body need after the exercise. Sleeping time is the time when you get to relax and let your body do the fixing up and repair work that it needs to keep you healthy.

Optimal sleep is going to be critical for any person who spends their time exercising on a regular basis. During the time that you sleep, your body is going to produce Growth Hormone; this is the hormone that holds a lot of responsibility for growing tissue and getting it repaired. If you do not get the sleep that you are supposed to or you skip out on it, the body is not able to produce this hormone and you will not be able to produce this hormone. This will all mean that you are not getting the recovery that your body needs and injury is much more likely.

Here are some tips that you can follow in order to get the best sleep that is possible when you are working out hard:

1. Go to bed early—yes, this may be a little bit difficult if you are used to staying up late or you have a lot of other things that you need to get through for the day. But you should make sure that you are getting in enough sleep in order to allow the body to rest and recover. Pick an early bed time and stick with it.

2. Avoid distractions—you need to avoid distractions as much as possible. Do not keep a TV in your room and keep noises to a minimum. These distractions are going to keep you awake or make it more difficult to get into the deep sleep that you need. If there are things outside of your control that keep you awake, such as a dog barking or neighbors who like to be outside late at night talking, consider getting something that can make white noise. Something like some soft and peaceful music or the static from a radio will be able to work for this.

3. Keep the room dark—when you have the room dark, it is easier to avoid distractions and get to sleep like you would need. You will also find that it is easier to get into a deeper sleep if you keep the room dark.

4. Be comfortable—it is not easy to fall asleep or stay asleep if you are not able to be as comfortable as possible. Pick out some pj's that

you like and feel soft, pick the blankets that you like, and get your mattress and pillow to be just the right softness or firmness so that you can be very comfortable. This will make it easier for you to fall asleep right away when your head hits the pillow.

5. Keep the room a little cool—finding the right temperature in order to fall asleep can be difficult. If you have the room too hot and you will be sweating and staying up for most of the night. On the other hand, if you keep it too cold, you will be shivering and up all night too. It is usually recommended that you keep the room a little bit cool though because this is able to promote better sleep. Setting the thermostat somewhere between 65 to 70 degrees is best for sleep and you can use a blanket to keep warmer if you like.

6. Glass of milk—warm up a little bit of milk to help you get into a deeper sleep. This has a calming and soothing effect on the body and can help you to get drowsy before going down. You might also want to consider a glass of water in order to get hydrated before dozing off.

These are just a few of the ideas that you can do to help your body get to sleep and feel the very best that it can during recovery.

Do Not Overtrain

When you are working out, you need to make sure that you are not overtraining one muscle or muscle group. If you do this, the recovery process is going to be pretty much impossible. You should have developed a workout plan that is smart and which will slowly work out the whole body over time rather than just one area to start with. If you are doing excessive exercises or heavy training each time that you work out, or if you are limiting your rest days, you will not be able to get the gains that you want out of the work out and you will make it difficult to recover the muscles, which results in injuries.

When you are making an exercise plan, you should make sure that you are separating out the workouts. Perhaps you can do a day of cardio and then a day of weight training. Or you can do a day of upper body and a day of lower body. Add in there a couple of rest days as well so the muscles can have a break. This helps to give all of the muscles a few days of rest so that they do not over train and become sore and prone to injury.

Use Visualization and Meditation

And for the final idea for preparing for the recovery, you should choose to use forms of visualization and meditation in order to reach your goals. If you are able to add in a type of mental practice to the routine, you are sure to see a lot of benefits to your results. This allows you to reach a calm and clear attitude about the workout and can reduce your reactivity and anxiety after a workout. This can help you also to learn how the mind works and when you understand this more, you will find that it is much easier to make your thoughts clear and get through the workout.

Most athletes will spend some time working on meditation or other visualization techniques in order to calm down the mind and get it on the track that is needed in order to work as well as possible. If you are interested in using meditation, here are a few things to keep in mind in order to do it properly:

1. Find a quiet place---you need to find a quiet place where you can be alone with your thoughts and not have to worry about anyone who is bothering you. You can find a quiet room or just a little corner where you can be alone with your thoughts for at least 15 minutes. This might be hard sometimes, but make sure to tell everyone around you that you are busy and ask that they leave you in peace for a short time.

2. Get comfortable—you will find that meditation is almost impossible if you are not able to get comfortable in the process. You should sit on the floor and have your legs crossed and your back straight in order to encourage the flow of energy through the body. If you are not able to sit on the

floor because of pain or it is not comfortable, it is fine to do this in a chair as well as long as you sit up straight and concentrate on posture.

3. Concentrate on breathing—take in slow breathes and let them go slowly as well. You want to be able to control the breathing that you are doing so that it is nice and steady. Often people will be breathing hard and all over the place, especially when you have been working out, and you will not be able to relax and let go of the anxiety with this uneven breathing. Take in the deep and slow breaths in order to get the heart rate down and in the place where you need it to be for relaxation.

4. Clear your head—while you are concentrating on the breathing, you should be able to feel your thoughts and your emotions just melt away into peace. If this is a little difficult for you, do not worry. Worrying is just going to make you upset and ruin the meditation experience. Everyone has some trouble with clearing out their minds and simply concentrating on their breathing so it is normal if this takes you some time to figure out. Just lead your mind back to the breathing and soon you will get the hang of it.

These are just some of the simple steps that you should take in order to do meditation. If you are interested in using this method in order to relax your mind and get it ready for the next workout, then you should take a look into some of the different forms of meditation to get a good idea of what might work for you.

These are ten of the best things that you will be able to do after a workout. They are meant to help get your mind in the right frame to get going, to help your muscles and body to get the nutrients that they need, and to help you through the whole recovery process when you are done so you can continue to get the benefits that you are looking for rather than getting an injury or hurting your body in the process. Give a few of them a try and be amazed at how much quicker recovery can be and how effective you can become with your workouts.

Conclusion

Everyone is going to have their own routine for getting a workout as well as their own reason for wanting to get to the gym. But no matter the personal reasons that might be your motivation, it is important that you follow some of the tips in this book, both for before the work out and for the recovery period after the work out. They are meant to help you in so many ways. You will find that your work out is much more efficient if you are able to stretch, stay hydrated, eat right, and follow the other tips that are presented in the first chapter. You will also find that recovery time is much easier and faster and that you are going to be less prone to injuries if you follow the great ideas that are listed in the second chapter. Give a few of them a try and see how great your next work out can be!

Thank you for reading my book. If you enjoyed this book and gained some value then I need your help; please take a moment to leave a review.

Dean Lacy